THE IMPACT OF TECHNOLOGY ON HEALTH CARE

UNDERSTANDING HEALTHCARE IN THE NEW WORLD

CYRIL LAKES

Contents

CHAPTER ONE

INTRODUCTION

Technology has had a revolutionary effect on healthcare, changing the way services are provided, accessed, and experienced. Technological developments in the healthcare business have brought in a new era of efficiency, accessibility, and individualized care. Examples of these innovations include wearable gadgets, artificial intelligence, and electronic health records and telemedicine.

This introduction examines the significant impacts of technology on healthcare, emphasizing significant developments, difficulties, and prospects for the provision of healthcare in the future. Healthcare practitioners can improve population health, improve patient outcomes, and spur innovation in healthcare delivery models by utilizing state-of-the-art technologies.

We will learn about the various ways that technological advancements are changing the face of modern medicine, empowering patients, and altering the patient-provider dynamic as we dig deeper into the effects of technology on healthcare.

The quick development of medical technologies

The quick development of technology in the healthcare sector has completely changed the way that medical services are provided, accessed, and experienced. Numerous technical advancements, such as wearable technology, telemedicine, artificial intelligence (AI), digital health solutions, and genetic medicine, have come together to promote this development. An outline of how these developments are changing healthcare can be found here:

Digital Health Solutions: The emergence of digital health solutions has simplified administrative procedures, boosted care coordination, and raised patient participation. Examples of these solutions include electronic health records (EHRs), health applications, and patient portals. These digital tools make it easier for medical professionals to obtain patient data, help patients communicate with one another, and provide people the power to actively manage their own health.

Artificial Intelligence (AI) and Machine Learning: By allowing clinical decision support systems, customized medicine, and predictive analytics, AI-powered technologies are transforming healthcare. Large volumes of medical data can be analyzed by machine learning algorithms, which can also be used to spot trends and provide insights to help with illness management, diagnosis, and treatment planning. Applications of AI include precision medicine, virtual health assistants, medication development, and interpretation of medical imaging.

Telemedicine and Remote Monitoring: In underdeveloped areas or during public health emergencies, telemedicine platforms and remote monitoring technology have increased access to healthcare services. Patients can manage chronic diseases from the comfort of their homes, obtain specialized expertise, and receive prompt care with the help of virtual consultations, digital health platforms, and remote monitoring of vital signs.

Wearable Technology and Remote Patient Monitoring: Health measurements, such as heart rate, activity level, and glucose levels, can be continuously monitored with wearable technology, which includes fitness trackers, smartwatches, and medical wearables. These gadgets improve the lives of people with chronic illnesses by enabling proactive health management, early abnormality identification, and remote patient monitoring.

Personalized healthcare approaches that are based on an individual's distinct genetic composition have been made possible by advancements in genomics and molecular diagnostics. Precision medicine initiatives, genetic testing for illness risk assessment, and targeted medicines based on genetic profiles are made possible by genomic sequencing technology, which also contribute to more efficient and individualized treatment plans.

Healthcare Robotics and Automation: By automating tedious tasks, increasing surgical precision, and improving patient outcomes, robotics and automation technologies are transforming the delivery of healthcare. Examples of how robotics is being used into different areas of healthcare to increase effectiveness and patient care include automated pharmacy systems, robotic exoskeletons, and surgical robots.

Blockchain and Health Information Exchange: Blockchain technology has the potential to improve data integrity in healthcare systems, enable interoperability, and securely store and share sensitive health data. Blockchain-based systems improve privacy and trust in healthcare transactions by facilitating safe data transparency, patient consent management, and the transmission of health information.

Virtual and Augmented Reality (VR/AR): Immersion therapy, patient education, and medical training are some of the uses of VR/AR technologies in the healthcare industry. In a risk-free setting, medical personnel can rehearse complex procedures with VR/AR simulations, while patients can benefit from immersive experiences that aid in pain management, anxiety reduction, and rehabilitation.

All things considered, the swift progress of technology in the healthcare sector is revolutionizing the field, spurring creativity, optimizing patient results, and elevating the efficacy and efficiency of healthcare provision.

Technology has the ability to improve healthcare, provide access to high-quality treatment, and enable people to live healthier lives in the digital age as it develops.

Patient Management

The use of technology in healthcare has transformed patient care and resulted in notable gains in effectiveness, accessibility, and quality. Technology is changing patient care in the following ways:

Improved Access to Care: Patients, especially those who live in rural or underserved areas, now have easier access to healthcare thanks to technology. Through the use of telemedicine platforms, patients can consult with medical professionals from a distance, eliminating the need for travel and facilitating access to medical knowledge wherever they may be.

Better Communication and Collaboration: Digital health solutions, like secure messaging platforms and electronic health records (EHRs), help healthcare providers communicate and work together more effectively, resulting in more patient-centered and coordinated care. Interoperable electronic health record systems facilitate the easy exchange of patient data between various healthcare environments, guaranteeing treatment continuity and lowering medical mistakes.

Personalized medicine: New developments in artificial intelligence, data analytics, and genomics make it possible to provide patients with individualized care. Healthcare professionals can customize treatment plans and interventions to each patient, maximizing benefits and minimizing side effects, by evaluating genetic, clinical, and lifestyle data.

Remote Monitoring and Chronic Disease Management: Wearable devices and remote monitoring technologies allow for continuous monitoring of patients' vital signs and health parameters outside of typical healthcare settings. This enables early detection of health abnormalities, proactive intervention, and better management of chronic conditions such as diabetes, hypertension, and heart disease.

Patient Engagement and Empowerment: Digital health tools empower patients to actively participate in their healthcare journey. Patient portals, mobile apps, and wearable devices provide patients with access to their health information, appointment scheduling, medication reminders, and educational resources, fostering greater engagement, self-management, and adherence to treatment plans.

Streamlined Clinical Workflows: Technology streamlines clinical workflows and administrative processes, reducing paperwork, minimizing duplication of efforts, and improving efficiency in healthcare delivery. Automated appointment scheduling, electronic prescribing, and telehealth platforms streamline administrative tasks, allowing healthcare providers to focus more time on patient care.

Improved Safety and Quality of Care: Technology enhances patient safety and quality of care through tools such as clinical decision support systems, medication reconciliation software, and barcode medication administration. These systems help minimize prescription errors, identify potential drug interactions, and assure adherence to evidence-based guidelines, leading to safer and more effective care delivery.

Healthcare Robotics and Surgical Innovation: Robotics and automation technologies are altering surgical methods and patient outcomes. Surgical robots offer minimally invasive surgeries with greater precision and faster recovery times, while robotic-assisted rehabilitation equipment improve mobility and functional outcomes for patients recuperating from accidents or surgeries.

Patient Privacy and Data Security: Technology plays a significant role in ensuring patient privacy and data security. Strict protocols, encryption technologies, and access restrictions are developed to protect sensitive health information contained in electronic health records and exchanged across digital channels, assuring compliance with privacy rules such as HIPAA.

Overall, the impact of technology on patient care in healthcare is considerable, driving advances in accessibility, quality, safety, and patient engagement. By leveraging technology efficiently, healthcare practitioners may deliver more personalized, efficient, and effective care, eventually improving health outcomes and enhancing the patient experience.

Diagnosis and Treatment

The impact of technology on healthcare has transformed both the diagnosis and treatment of medical diseases, leading to developments that boost accuracy, efficiency, and effectiveness. Here's how technology is revolutionizing diagnosis and treatment in healthcare:

Diagnosis:

Medical Imaging: Advanced imaging technologies such as magnetic resonance imaging (MRI), computed tomography (CT), and ultrasound have substantially increased diagnostic capabilities. These imaging technologies provide precise views of inside structures, enabling healthcare providers to discover irregularities, diagnose diseases, and design suitable treatment plans.

Artificial Intelligence (AI) in Diagnostics: AI-powered diagnostic systems utilize machine learning algorithms to assess medical pictures, laboratory data, and patient information. These AI systems can discover trends, identify anomalies, and assist healthcare providers in identifying illnesses with more accuracy and efficiency, leading to speedier treatment decisions and improved patient outcomes.

CHAPTER TWO

Genomic Sequencing: Genetic variants linked to diseases and ailments can be identified by analyzing an individual's genetic code using genomic sequencing technologies. Based on each person's distinct genetic composition, genetic testing and personalized genomic medicine enable more accurate diagnoses, focused medicines, and customized treatment regimens.

Point-of-Care Testing: Quick diagnostic testing at the bedside or in unconventional settings is made possible by advancements in point-of-care testing technologies. Point-of-care testing for metabolic disorders, infectious infections, and chronic problems yield answers quickly, allowing for early diagnosis and patient management that is appropriate.

Wearable technology and remote monitoring: These two trends together enable ongoing patient health measurements to be tracked even when patients are not in medical facilities. Vital signs, blood glucose levels, exercise levels, and other health metrics can all be tracked by these devices, which makes it possible to identify health issues early and to provide remote diagnosis and treatment.

Therapy:

Precision Medicine: These methods customize treatment plans for each patient according to their distinct clinical, genetic, and lifestyle traits.

Better patient outcomes are made possible by tailored medications that are more effective and have fewer side effects than conventional treatments thanks to genomic sequencing, biomarker testing, and molecular diagnostics.

Robotics-Assisted Surgery: By improving surgical control, dexterity, and precision, robotics-assisted surgical devices enable less invasive treatments with smaller incisions and quicker recovery periods. Surgeons can execute intricate surgeries with increased precision and fewer difficulties thanks to robotic surgery platforms, which enhance patient outcomes and shorten hospital stays.

Drug Discovery and Development: Computational modeling, high-throughput screening, and virtual drug design are some of the ways that technology is accelerating these processes. Large-scale datasets are analyzed by AI algorithms to find possible medication candidates, forecast their safety and efficacy profiles, and customize treatment plans. This process expedites the discovery of novel medicines and individualized care plans.

Virtual care and telemedicine: Digital health tools, video conferencing, and secure messaging are used by telemedicine systems to facilitate remote consultations, diagnosis, and treatment administration. Virtual care services increase patient access to healthcare, especially for those living in underserved or rural locations. They also make follow-up treatment and timely intervention possible without requiring in-person visits.

Medical Devices and Therapies: Patient outcomes and quality of life are enhanced by technological advancements in medical devices and therapies. Targeted medicines, gene therapies, and immunotherapies provide new choices for treating cancer and other complicated diseases, while advanced prostheses, implantable devices, and medical implants help patients with disabilities or injuries regain function and movement.

All things considered, technology has a revolutionary effect on healthcare diagnosis and treatment, resulting in more precise diagnoses, individualized treatment plans, and better patient outcomes. Healthcare professionals can improve patient outcomes and healthcare delivery quality by efficiently utilizing technological innovations to give more precise, efficient, and patient-centered treatment.

Information Administration

Because data management makes it possible to store, analyze, and use enormous volumes of health-related information, it is essential to understanding how technology is affecting healthcare. The following are some ways that data management is helping to transform healthcare:

Electronic Health Records (EHRs): EHR systems make it easier to store and manage patient health information digitally, including prescriptions, test results, treatment plans, and medical histories. By giving healthcare practitioners access to complete and current information, electronic health records (EHRs) improve care coordination, expedite data access, and aid in clinical decision-making.

Health Information interchange (HIE) and Interoperability: The main goals of data management programs are to facilitate the smooth interchange of health information between various healthcare systems and environments. Health information exchange (HIE) networks allow medical professionals to securely share patient data, which enhances patient safety, care coordination, and minimizes test duplication.

Big Data Analytics: By analyzing vast amounts of healthcare data, sophisticated analytics tools and methodologies are able to identify patterns and insights that guide population health management, clinical decision-making, and healthcare policy. The utilization of big data analytics facilitates evidence-based practices and quality improvement programs by enabling predictive modeling, risk stratification, and pattern recognition in patient outcomes.

Clinical Decision Support Systems (CDSS): Assisting healthcare providers in real time at the point of care, data management systems include clinical decision support capabilities into electronic health records. Clinical Decision Support Systems (CDSS) use patient data, medical literature, and best practice standards to help physicians diagnose illnesses, choose the best course of therapy, and avoid medical errors.

Data Security and Privacy: To guard against unauthorized access, breaches, and abuse of sensitive patient information, data management in the healthcare industry places a high priority on security and privacy safeguards. Ensuring the confidentiality, integrity, and availability of healthcare data is crucial for protecting patient privacy and trust. This can be achieved by robust data encryption, access restrictions, and compliance with regulatory requirements like HIPAA.

Population Health Management: To uncover health inequities, track illness patterns, and focus interventions, data management strategies aggregate and analyze data from many sources. This helps to support population health initiatives. Healthcare organizations can use population health management platforms to stratify populations, monitor results, and apply preventative care methods in order to lower healthcare costs and improve overall health outcomes.

Research and Innovation: By granting access to extensive, longitudinal datasets for epidemiological studies, clinical trials, and outcomes research, healthcare data management fosters research and innovation in the field of medicine. The pace of discovery and innovation in healthcare is accelerated by the collaboration of researchers, physicians, and industry stakeholders made possible via research databases, data repositories, and data sharing platforms.

Patient Empowerment and Engagement: Data management programs provide patients the ability to take charge of their own care, maintain and access their health information, and take part in collaborative decision-making. Transparency, autonomy, and self-management are encouraged by patient portals, mobile health applications, and personal health records, which allow users to access test results, make appointments, and contact with medical professionals.

All things considered, efficient data management is necessary to fully utilize technology in healthcare, support evidence-based procedures, enhance clinical results, and improve patient satisfaction. Healthcare companies may enhance the quality of care provided, stimulate innovation, and improve the health of both individuals and communities by utilizing data-driven insights and technologies.

Patient Involvement and Instruction

The impact of technology on healthcare is mostly dependent on patient participation and education, which enable people to take an active role in their own health management and decision-making. The following are some ways that technology in healthcare promotes patient education and engagement:

Health Information Portals and Websites: Thanks to technology, people can now obtain trustworthy and current information about medical issues, available treatments, and preventive care through online portals and websites. These platforms include interactive tools, articles, videos, and educational resources to help patients make educated decisions and gain knowledge.

Applications for Mobile Health: Apps for mobile health provide easy-to-use and accessible platforms for self-management, health monitoring, and patient education. In order to promote involvement and accountability in their care, patients can use health apps to track symptoms, medication adherence, and vital signs. They can also access educational content on a range of health-related topics and receive individualized health recommendations.

Telehealth and Virtual Consultations: By using video conferencing, secure messaging, and telemedicine apps, telehealth platforms enable patients and healthcare professionals to have virtual visits and remote consultations. Virtual consultations improve patient involvement and lower barriers to healthcare access by providing patients with easy access to follow-up treatment, specialist consultations, and medical advice from the comfort of their homes.

Patient portals and personal health records (PHRs): These online tools give patients safe access to, viewing of, and management of their medical records. Transparency, communication, and active patient involvement are encouraged by patient portals, which enable users to access medical histories, request medication refills, connect with healthcare practitioners, and review lab results.

Wearable Technology and Remote Monitoring: Patients can monitor their health measurements and activities in real-time with wearable technology, including smartwatches, fitness trackers, and medical wearables. Through the provision of feedback, insights, and reminders, these devices enable patients to take proactive measures towards improving their health outcomes by promoting healthy behaviors, self-monitoring, and adherence to treatment plans.

Online Support Communities and Social Media: Thanks to technology, people can connect with others going through comparable medical issues, share their stories, and offer advice and support. Online support communities and social media groups are made possible. Engaging in virtual communities offers patients a feeling of community, helpful guidance, and emotional support all of which promote peer support and self-determination.

Gamification and Behavior Change Interventions: To encourage and involve patients in embracing healthy behaviors, gamification strategies and behavior change interventions are applied in health apps and digital platforms. Patients are encouraged to set objectives, monitor their progress, and adopt healthier lifestyles using gamified challenges, prizes, and incentives. This improves motivation, adherence, and long-term health results.

Educational Videos and Interactive Tools: Thanks to technology, patients can be more actively engaged in learning about intricate medical ideas and procedures by watching educational videos, animations, and interactive tools. In order to improve comprehension, retention, and engagement in patient education, multimedia resources include visual explanations, demonstrations, and simulations.

All things considered, technology is essential for encouraging patient involvement and education in the medical field and enabling people to take an active role in their own health and wellbeing. Through the utilization of technology-driven tools and platforms, healthcare providers can augment patient education, cultivate self-management abilities, and ultimately boost health results and patient contentment.

Healthcare Personnel and Education

The workforce and training are also impacted by technology's influence on healthcare, which changes how medical personnel provide treatment, pick up new skills, and adjust to changing procedures. Here are some ways that technology is changing the training and workforce in healthcare:

Digital Skills and Competencies: Healthcare workers must become proficient users of technology-enabled tools and platforms and acquire digital literacy. In order to guarantee the efficient use of technology in clinical practice, training programs and continuing education initiatives concentrate on improving digital skills, including familiarity with electronic health records (EHRs), telemedicine platforms, and medical devices.

Training in Telemedicine and Virtual Care: Programs in telemedicine and virtual care educate medical professionals to provide care via secure messaging, video consultations, and telehealth platforms from a distance. In order to enable providers to provide high-quality treatment in virtual environments, training emphasizes communication skills, virtual evaluation procedures, and adherence to telemedicine norms and laws.

Simulation-Based Training: By utilizing augmented reality (AR) and virtual reality (VR) technologies, simulation-based training offers medical practitioners immersive learning opportunities to practice surgical techniques, clinical skills, and emergency situations. With the use of virtual simulations, trainers may perfect their abilities, make better decisions, and increase patient safety in a realistic and safe environment.

Artificial Intelligence (AI) in Healthcare Training: To improve patient care, diagnosis, and treatment planning, healthcare professionals receive training on how to use AI-powered technologies and clinical decision support systems. In order to maximize results and efficiency, training programs concentrate on comprehending AI algorithms, interpreting insights produced by AI, and incorporating AI technology into clinical processes.

Technology facilitates communication and information exchange among healthcare workers from various disciplines and contexts, which in turn fosters multidisciplinary collaboration and team-based care. Interprofessional training programs provide a strong emphasis on collaboration, communication techniques, and collaborative practice models, which help healthcare teams to effectively collaborate and provide coordinated treatment.

Health informatics and Data Analytics Training: Data analytics, health informatics, and data-driven decision-making are all covered in healthcare worker training. Healthcare workers can enhance patient care, population health management, and healthcare delivery procedures by learning how to evaluate healthcare data, interpret clinical outcomes, and apply data insights from training programs.

Professional Development and Continuing Education: Healthcare workers can stay current on emerging trends, best practices, and technology developments by taking advantage of professional development opportunities and continuing education programs. Initiatives for lifelong learning facilitate continuous competency maintenance, knowledge acquisition, and skill development, allowing healthcare workers to adjust to changes in practice and technology throughout the course of their careers.

Healthcare workforce training encompasses ethical and regulatory aspects pertaining to the use of technology in the healthcare industry. These aspects include patient privacy, data security, informed consent, and adherence to healthcare standards like HIPAA. Training programs have a strong emphasis on using technology-enabled tools and platforms with professionalism, discretion, and ethical decision-making.

All things considered, implementing technology-enabled training programs is crucial to enabling the medical staff to fully utilize technology in the delivery of healthcare. Healthcare companies may make sure that healthcare workers have the information, skills, and competencies required to deliver safe, efficient, and patient-centered care in the digital era by investing in workforce development and training programs that use technology.

CHAPTER THREE

Upcoming Patterns

Innovation, new trends, and changing patient and provider demands are all driving changes in the way that technology is affecting healthcare. The following upcoming trends have the potential to influence how healthcare technology develops:

Artificial Intelligence (AI) and Machine Learning: These two fields will remain crucial to the healthcare industry, as they enable clinical decision support systems, personalized treatment, and predictive analytics. Large-scale healthcare data will be analyzed by AI algorithms to find trends, forecast results, and improve treatment strategies, resulting in more accurate diagnosis and customized treatments.

The integration of telemedicine and virtual care into healthcare delivery models is anticipated to increase, providing easy and easily accessible choices for remote consultations, monitoring, and follow-up care. In order to increase patient outcomes and increase access to healthcare services, virtual care platforms will make use of technology including digital health tools, video conferencing, and remote monitoring.

Wearable technology and remote monitoring: As these technologies develop, it will be possible to continuously monitor patients' health-related behaviors and indicators. In order to offer real-time insights, early health abnormality identification, and individualized interventions for chronic disease management and preventive care, these devices will interface with AI algorithms.

Precision Medicine and Genomics: Utilizing molecular diagnostics, biomarker testing, and genetic sequencing to customize treatment plans for each patient, precision medicine techniques will keep developing. Targeted medicines, immunotherapies, and gene editing approaches that address the underlying genetic causes of diseases will be made possible by advances in genomics, providing more effective and individualized therapy options.

Blockchain and Health Data Security: The security, interoperability, and patient privacy of health data will all be improved by the growing adoption of blockchain technology. Blockchain-based systems will make it possible to interchange data amongst healthcare stakeholders, securely share and store private health information, and guarantee the integrity and transparency of healthcare transactions.

Technologies such as augmented reality (AR) and virtual reality (VR) will be used in patient education, surgical simulation, medical training, and therapeutic treatments. Healthcare workers will be able to practice difficult procedures through immersive experiences, improve patient comprehension of medical diagnoses and treatments, and provide immersive therapies for pain management and rehabilitation.

Internet of Medical Things (IoMT): This network of interconnected medical equipment, sensors, and wearables will keep growing as it links them to the internet for data gathering, analysis, and remote monitoring. IoMT devices will make proactive interventions for early disease identification and management, predictive analytics, and personalized health monitoring possible.

Healthcare Robotics and Automation: As robotics and automation technologies develop, they will improve patient care delivery, surgical techniques, and clinical processes. Automation in healthcare settings will be enhanced by robotic-assisted surgery systems, robotic exoskeletons, and automated care assistants;

administrative work and data management procedures will be streamlined by robotic process automation (RPA).

These emerging patterns in the use of technology in healthcare provide promising chances to improve patient care, achieve better results, and change the way healthcare is delivered. Healthcare companies may fully utilize technology to address healthcare concerns, improve efficiency, and promote better health outcomes for both individuals and communities by embracing technological breakthroughs and innovation.

Summary

In summary, technology has a significant and wide-ranging impact on the healthcare sector, changing every facet of the business from patient care and staff development to diagnosis and treatment. Technological developments have completely changed the way healthcare is delivered, increasing patient and provider access, effectiveness, and quality of care while equipping them with the knowledge and resources they need to improve patient outcomes.

The following are some salient points of how technology is affecting healthcare:

Enhanced Convenience and Access: The utilization of telemedicine, virtual care, and remote monitoring technology has resulted in an increase in the availability of healthcare services, especially for underprivileged and isolated populations. With the convenience of their homes, patients may now obtain prompt care, consultations, and monitoring, which lowers barriers to care and enhances patient outcomes.

Improved Diagnosis and Treatment: Genomic medicine, artificial intelligence, and advanced imaging technologies have completely changed how diseases are diagnosed and treated. Thanks to precision medicine initiatives that are based on the unique genetic profiles and clinical requirements of each patient, healthcare providers can now make more precise diagnoses, customize treatment strategies, and maximize outcomes.

Patient Empowerment and Engagement: Patients are given the ability to actively take part in their healthcare journey, obtain health information, and collaborate with their healthcare providers on decisions through the use of technology-enabled tools and platforms. Healthy lifestyles, self-management, and treatment plan adherence are encouraged by wearable technology, mobile health apps, and patient portals.

Efficiency and Innovation: Technology promotes innovation in healthcare delivery models, improves communication and collaboration among healthcare workers, and streamlines clinical operations. Platforms for telemedicine, data analytics tools, and electronic health records enhance care coordination, boost productivity, and promote evidence-based practices.

Education and Training: Technology makes it easier for healthcare workers to receive continuing education and training, giving them access to digital skills, telemedicine knowledge, and competency with AI-powered technologies. Healthcare personnel can stay current on emerging trends and best practices in healthcare delivery with the help of online learning platforms, virtual reality simulations, and simulation-based training.

Data Management and Security: Ensuring the confidentiality, integrity, and accessibility of healthcare data is made possible by strong data management systems and security measures. Interoperable EHR systems, blockchain technology, and health information exchange networks allow for the safe sharing and exchange of patient data while protecting against privacy issues and data breaches.

Prospective Developments and Prospects: New developments in the fields of precision medicine, telemedicine, AI-powered diagnostics, and health robotics present promising avenues for enhancing patient outcomes and revolutionizing healthcare delivery. By embracing innovation and leveraging technological advancements, healthcare organizations can address healthcare challenges, drive efficiency, and advance the goal of providing high-quality, patient-centered care.

In conclusion, technology is having a revolutionary effect on healthcare, paving the way for a time when treatment is more easily obtainable, customized, and effective than in the past. Healthcare stakeholders may keep promoting positive change, bettering health outcomes, and enhancing the general well-being of people and communities worldwide by embracing technological breakthroughs and innovation.

THE END